THE COMPLETE DIABETIC COOKBOOK FOR BEGINNERS 2024

1500+ Days of Super Easy and Delicious Recipes to Manage Type 2 Diabetes, Pre-Diabetes and Newly Diagnosed With a 21-Day Meal Plan

TERESA R. THOMAS

Table of Contents

INTRODUCTION

I realize it's terrifying. Being diagnosed with diabetes might be overwhelming at first. Many people believe they have diabetes, but it's only confirmed by a doctor's official diagnosis.

I felt gut-punched when I walked out of the doctor's office after learning I had diabetes. I suspected I had it and had certain symptoms, but until the 'incident' that prompted me to see a doctor, I only considered the possibility briefly.

Maybe it was diabetes, maybe it wasn't. It was easy to put off the reality until tomorrow. I will deal with it later.

After 'later', I sat on my sofa with my springer spaniel by my side, staring out the window. She saw I was angry.

Was 'upset' the right word? I was experiencing several feelings, including sorrow, remorse, bewilderment, anxiety, and loss. And did I mention fear?

What was I planning to do? Take the meds, yes. I was uncertain about it. My doctor recommended solutions for managing my type 2 diabetes. I dislike having to adhere to a strict diet. Why can't I eat anything I want and still be healthy? I needed to exercise more (what else is new? I've struggled with this issue since childhood.

Diabetes runs in my family. I should not have been startled by the diagnosis. But it always felt like it was at arm's length, that it was never my concern, but always theirs, since they were the sick ones.

Surprise. It was now mine, and I needed to accept responsibility for it.

I wallowed in my own misery for a few weeks.

When my pals asked whether I was alright, I didn't answer the door and instead texted them some excuse for being out or in the shower. I decided to be honest. One of my voice messages was heard clearly.

"Jo, I understand you're worried. I understand your desire to avoid the matter, but it is unavoidable. I spoke with your aunt, who informed me that you had seen a diabetic specialist. It's not hard to arrive at a decision. Could we perhaps enjoy an afternoon together? I'd want to share my approach to dealing with challenges and provide tips on how to cope with them, regardless of severity or fear. "Please call me!"

Did Olivia have diabetes? Despite our friendship dating back to college, I had no idea. Although she was more active than me, she did not seem to be a gym junkie. Her diet seems healthy. She ate both healthy foods and treats, albeit not as much as I did. Perhaps she might help me find a way out of my current situation.

Olivia and I met for tea at a small sidewalk café and spent two hours discussing how she rearranged her life to accommodate her illness. She referred to it as something other than an illness, which made me feel more at peace.

She presented me with numbers that prompted reflection. Type 2 diabetes affects many individuals, and it's not only my responsibility. American advertising promotes unhealthy eating habits, including preservatives, sugar, and other non-nutrients that may lead to pre-diabetes. In recent years, more children, teenagers, and young adults than ever before have been diagnosed with this disease, which affects both the young and the elderly.

I have type 2 diabetes, which prevents natural pancreatic insulin from entering cells and converting carbohydrates into energy. Fat within cells hinders insulin function, resulting in unhealthy blood sugar and glucose levels. If not addressed, excessive levels may lead to weight gain and damage cells that protect the heart, blood, brain, and vision.

It may cause symptoms such as fatigue, dizziness, nausea, and shortness of breath.

During our conversation, I recall my doctor suggesting I start taking insulin due to my bad health history. We would manage the dosage to ensure I was not taking more than necessary.

Poor health history? What exactly did it mean? Olivia assumed that meant I ate badly and didn't exercise. However, she suggested that with simple lifestyle changes, I may perhaps eliminate the need for insulin.

I was up for it!

This is a collection of my two-year journey learning about type 2 diabetes, experimenting with a plant-based diet, eating healthily, and altering my lifestyle, including the dreaded exercise!

I stopped using insulin and now work as a dietitian. I have been a dietitian for eight years. And I feel fantastic!

If you aren't interested in altering your lifestyle, you probably wouldn't be reading this book.

And I appreciate your boldness. I understand how difficult it may be to feel compelled to change, rather than desiring to. Embracing change may help you overcome minor obstacles.

As you go through this book, you'll:

- Learn about diabetes and how to manage it through diet and exercise.

- Learn how to recognize symptoms and distinguish between type 1 and type 2 diabetes.

- Learn how to regulate blood sugar levels, create a nutritious meal plate, and control portion sizes—access over 500 recipes.

As you gain control over your fear and anxiety, you will experience the outcomes above. Educating yourself and making lifestyle and nutritional adjustments may alleviate fears and anxieties.

Welcome to life with diabetes on your terms.

CHAPTER 1: BEFORE GETTING STARTED

The Basics of Diabetes

You may feel like a victim if you are diagnosed with diabetes unexpectedly. You may feel as if you have an uncontrollable inner evil you don't want to be associated with. And you are quite right in feeling this way.

Remember that you can live a fulfilling life even with diabetes. However, you must make certain changes and prioritize your own needs. You are the only one who will profit from your modifications, so take charge of your condition by making your own decisions.

Diabetes is unique in that it is a manageable condition. As you embark on your path, get support from your doctor, dietitian, nutritionist, diabetes educator, and pharmacist. By understanding the benefits of particular strategies, avoiding mistakes, and adapting to changes that enhance your health, you may live a fulfilling and healthy lifestyle on your terms.

Managing diabetes may require medicine to manage insulin levels. You may be able to wean off them or need to incorporate a dosage in your regular diet. Blood sugar levels will influence this. Maintaining a blood sugar level near to your goal might help avoid or postpone diabetes-related issues, which are a common source of anxiety for those diagnosed. We've all heard about the tragedies.

I won't speak about how simple it will be or how you can overlook the obvious; you can't. Diabetes may be manageable with regular blood sugar checks and adjustments (knowing what can be altered is crucial).

Some individuals avoid making required adjustments to enhance their well-being and health. I understand that. You are unique and can make little changes to improve your health, appearance, and ability to live a fulfilling life.

Diabetes is caused by high blood sugar levels, whether due to insulin insufficiency or resistance. If left untreated, it may overwhelm your kidneys and leak into your urine. Diabetes may cause blindness, renal failure, stroke, and heart attacks due to the breakdown of tissue caused by high blood sugar levels.

High blood sugar may damage nerves, leading to neuropathy. Damage symptoms include numbness, tingling, and discomfort. Poor circulation may cause loss of sensation in the limbs, leading to poor healing and amputations.

Diabetes prevalence has risen in the previous 30 years, with over 20 million Americans diagnosed with type 1 (5%-10%) or type 2 (90%-95%).

Knowing these facts may help you avoid future temptations. They had a significant impact on me. Ignoring these tiny but critical adjustments might lead to the same worry you had when initially diagnosed with diabetes. Ignoring warnings and causing harm may reinforce your dread.

Type 2 diabetes occurs when cells form a sticky material that resists insulin, making it difficult for them to ingest the glucose required for energy and cell regeneration.

Have you any clue what this gooey material is? It is fat. Plain and straightforward.

Type 1 diabetes may be managed by insulin regulation, which reconstructs insulin for cell utilization. Type 2 diabetes may be managed with drugs, but maintaining an active lifestyle and a healthy diet is the most effective and healthiest approach. You have power over both of these things.

Develop Good Habits

Here are important behaviors to cultivate for any stage of diabetes:

- Consume lots of water and avoid sugary beverages.

- Increase your vegetable intake and try new healthy foods.

- Create an enjoyable workout routine.

- Maintain daily blood sugar records;

- Identify and correct signs of high or low blood sugar;

- Take medication as prescribed;

- Monitor feet, eyes, and skin for potential symptoms;

- Properly store diabetic supplies and food (medications and meal ingredients) for optimal results;

- Exercise and a doctor-recommended program may help manage stress and anxiety.

As you learn new habits, it's important to have a support network to help you through any mistakes you may make. Find a companion to contact when feeling lost or anxious. They may be your lifeline for both health and sanity. Over time, this individual will become a trusted ally, creating a friendship worth cherishing for both parties.

CHAPTER 2: DESIGNING YOUR MENU

What Tips Do You Have For Preparing Delicious Meals?

- Fresh ingredients.

- Careful planning.

- Experience combining herbs and spices.

- Attractively presenting the dish.

If you agree on these basics, you've been paying attention to your meals, right? You can tell whether a meal is excellent or not. You've experienced both positive and negative outcomes.

You may believe it's difficult to enjoy healthy food since you've never tried it before. You probably assumed that was rabbit food.

I'm here to inform you that eating healthy doesn't have to be difficult, boring, or unpleasant, even if you dislike some items. Using the recommended components and preparation techniques will enhance the taste and intrigue of your dinners, save time, and allow for easy customization for a balanced and delightful diet.

Before preparing meals, it's important to understand the fundamentals of eating and why some foods are more enjoyable than others.

Nutrition and Diabetes

Foods are composed of three macronutrients: proteins, carbs, and fats. A nutrition label on a packaged food item lists components and their proportion of the daily recommended amount, as well as a breakdown of nutrients such as fiber, sugar, saturated and trans fats, and salt. The components used in the product are listed from highest to lowest percentages.

Diabetes is a significant health danger in America, with a 30% increase in cases and the 7th highest mortality rate.

Knowing the packaging contents is beneficial not just for what's inside, which is often processed and high in sugar, but also for what's missing. This is why you return most items to the shelf after reading their labels.

Recipes for a new diet often include two to five items.

The majority of the components are not often found in produce, meat, or baking sections.

Preservatives in processed food are commonly related to sugar or fructose syrups, which were formerly natural preservatives. This is due to the makers' demand for lengthy shelf life. Consuming chemical-laden processed foods has been linked to obesity and type 2 diabetes.

Let's move on from the negative and concentrate on the positive.

Proteins include meat, poultry, beans, nuts, eggs, shellfish, soy products, and seeds. Peas and beans are also considered vegetables. Proteins, whether lean or high in fat, should be carefully considered when planning your daily diet. Proteins, composed of amino acids, promote tissue growth, muscular strength, and blood health.

Carbohydrates, composed of sugars and starches, supply energy to cells, including the brain, the body's sole carbohydrate-dependent organ. The RDA for carb consumption is 130 grams per day for adults, although most eat between 220 and 330 grams for males and 180 to 230 grams for women. Carbohydrates may be found in starchy root vegetables, breads, cereals, fruits, and rice.

Fat is classified into four types: saturated fat, which is solid at room temperature and comes from animals; unsaturated fat, which is liquid at room temperature and comes from plants and may be further broken down into monounsaturated and polyunsaturated fat (olive oil, nuts, and seeds).

Fiber benefits our digestive system, blood, and organ health. Fiber prevents the accumulation of antioxidants and eliminates toxins and free radicals from the digestive system.

Water acts as a natural lubricant for all of our bodily functions.

Maintaining a high water intake is crucial since humans are 85% water. This is due to evaporation via perspiration, toxin removal (urine), and salt overload.

Learning about the functions of different foods will help you understand how they impact your body's systems and overall health.

Adding 3 portions of leafy greens to your diet can improve your vision, digestive health, and sense of taste.

Whole foods and plant-based diets may improve your senses, including taste, smell, and appreciation for flavor combinations.

It's as if a curtain is removed from your taste receptors, and almost every other system responds to your enhancements. Premium foods are the ideal fuel for your body.

Is it necessary to emphasize the benefits of a healthier diet on the skin? Restore suppleness, reduce wrinkles, increase elasticity, and achieve a young 'glow' from the inside.

How Much Should I Eat?

When planning your diet, aim for a daily calorie intake of 2000-2800. Consider varying food types and portion sizes. Consult your doctor to determine the appropriate calorie intake based on your activity level, age, and diabetes management plan. Several things may contribute to achieving the ideal body shape.

Balance your meals by including proteins, carbohydrates, and fat. A plant-based diet with whole grains provides a foundation for daily meals.

Portion guidelines for each meal should be approximately as follows:

- Include ½ plate of non-starchy veggies such as broccoli, green beans, asparagus, peppers, carrots, cucumbers, onions, and cauliflower.

- Consume ¼ plate of healthy protein sources, including shellfish, eggs, edamame, low-fat dairy and yogurt, chicken or turkey, tuna, beans, and tofu.

- ¼ plate carbs: berries, peas, lentils, healthy grains (no sugar), oats, and quinoa.

Using this blueprint, you may create a tasty supper with a variety of flavors.

This book's recipes allow for easy substitution of ingredients while maintaining the core cooking procedure, allowing for versatile meal options.

If you don't have potatoes, you may simply replace them with sweet potatoes, beets, or squash (zucchini or butternut) to create a unique meal. Experiment with different meal combinations!

To improve your dining experience and reduce your risk of diabetes, try several 'tricks' for enticing food tastes.

- Eat at the table instead of in front of the TV to avoid temptations. Eat slowly and digest each mouthful thoroughly. Allow at least 20 minutes to complete your meal. This is the time it takes your stomach to feel full.

- Drinking enough water is both beneficial to your health and calorie-free.

- Make healthy substitutions for favorite meals and cuisines.

- When cooking, include people and make it a 'party.'

- Shop with a full stomach to avoid harmful temptations.

- Read labels and educate yourself on the ingredients in pre-packaged meals.

- Don't feel like you have to 'clear' your plate. Keep baggies or plastic containers on hand to store leftovers.

- Serve smaller servings.

- Plate your meals on the kitchen counter, not at the table.

Follow the advice and guidelines. This approach not only lowers blood sugar levels and improves health, but also develops a lifelong capacity to monitor and control diabetes.

CHAPTER 3

Pantry and Craving Lists

Do you feel more comfortable arranging your meals now?

Are you confident in making the required changes for a fulfilling, healthy, and happy life?

Creating a healthy diet plan might be challenging, particularly when you don't have anything to eat. However, it's not impossible.

Here's a list of backup products to have on hand for unexpected weekends or a busy workweek.

Pantry List

Maintain a supply of these products on hand at all times. Use them as a major or auxiliary element in your meal. Don't simply eat 'carrots' or 'blueberries.' Create unique smoothies, omelets, and Asian bowls by mixing and matching ingredients. Keep nutritious snack options on hand, such as almonds, seeds, berries, or olives.

- Apple

- Raspberries

- Loganberries

- Strawberries

- Blueberries

- Wild salmon

- Haddock

- Tuna

- Swordfish

- Mackerel

- Avocados

- Dark chocolate (75% plus)

- Red onions

- Carrots

- Greek yogurt

- Oats

- Cinnamon

- Turmeric

- Leafy greens

- Garlic

- Flaxseed

- Nuts

- Olive oil

- Coconut oil

- Bell peppers

- Black coffee

- Green juice

CRAVINGS LIST

The dreaded 'craving' may disrupt an otherwise well-structured week. Knowing your bodily needs might help you remain on track and avoid bingeing.

These supplements are essential for our health, but they may be difficult to remember to take during holidays or hectic periods.

Keep a variety of food substitutes on hand to satisfy your cravings without overindulging. Providing alternatives for your ' munchies' helps your body acquire the necessary nutrients, fulfilling cravings and gradually reducing them.

CHAPTER 4

Breakfast Recipes

1 - Walnut and Oat Granola

Ingredients:

- 3 cups rolled oats

- 1 cup chopped walnuts

- 1/4 cup honey or maple syrup

- 1/4 cup coconut oil or vegetable oil

- 1/2 teaspoon cinnamon (optional)

- 1/4 teaspoon salt

- 1/2 cup dried fruits (such as raisins, cranberries, or apricots) (optional)

Preparation:

1. Preheat the oven to 300°F (150°C), and line a baking sheet with parchment paper.

2. In a large mixing bowl, combine the rolled oats and chopped walnuts.

3. In a small saucepan, heat the honey or maple syrup and coconut oil over low heat until melted and well combined. Stir in the cinnamon and salt.

4. Pour the honey or maple syrup mixture over the oats and walnuts, and stir until evenly coated.

5. Evenly distribute the mixture onto the prepared baking sheet.

6. Bake for 25-30 minutes, stirring halfway through, until the granola is golden brown and crisp.

7. Remove from the oven and let to cool fully on the baking sheet.

8. Once cooled, stir in the dried fruits if using.

9. Keep the granola in an airtight jar at room temperature for up to two weeks.

Nutritional Value:

- Serving size: 1/2 cup

- Calories: Approximately 250

- Total fat: 14g

- Saturated fat: 5g

- Cholesterol: 0mg

- Sodium: 60mg

- Total carbohydrates: 28g

- Dietary fiber: 4g

- Sugars: 10g

- Protein: 6g

Cooking Time: Approximately 25-30 minutes

2 - Crispy Pita with Canadian Bacon

Ingredients:

- 4 whole wheat pitas

- 8 slices Canadian bacon

- 1 cup shredded mozzarella cheese

- 1/2 cup marinara sauce

- 1/4 cup chopped fresh basil

- Olive oil, for brushing

- Salt and pepper to taste

Preparation:

1. Preheat your oven to 400°F (200°C).

2. Place the pitas on a baking sheet lined with parchment paper.

3. Brush the pitas lightly with olive oil on both sides.

4. Place two slices of Canadian bacon on each pita.

5. Spoon marinara sauce evenly over the Canadian bacon.

6. Sprinkle shredded mozzarella cheese over the marinara sauce.

7. Add salt and pepper to taste.

8. Bake in the preheated oven for 8-10 minutes, or until the cheese is melted and bubbly, and the edges of the pitas are crispy.

9. Remove from the oven and sprinkle chopped fresh basil over the top.

10. Slice into wedges and serve immediately.

Nutritional Value:

- Serving size: 1 crispy pita

- Calories: Approximately 280

- Total fat: 10g

- Saturated fat: 4g

- Cholesterol: 30mg

- Sodium: 620mg

- Total carbohydrates: 30g

- Dietary fiber: 3g

- Sugars: 2g

- Protein: 18g

Cooking Time: Approximately 8-10 minutes

3 - Coconut and Chia Pudding

Ingredients:

- 1/4 cup chia seeds

- 1 cup coconut milk (can use full-fat or light)

- 1 tablespoon maple syrup or honey (optional)

- 1/2 teaspoon vanilla extract

- Fresh fruit, coconut flakes, or nuts for topping (optional)

Preparation:

1. In a bowl, combine the chia seeds, coconut milk, maple syrup or honey (if using), and vanilla extract. Stir well to combine.

2. Cover the bowl and refrigerate for at least 2 hours or overnight, stirring occasionally. This causes the chia seeds to absorb the liquid and form a pudding-like consistency.

3. Once the pudding has thickened to your desired consistency, give it a final stir.

4. Divide the pudding into serving bowls or jars.

5. Top with fresh fruit, coconut flakes, or nuts if desired.

6. Serve chilled and enjoy!

Nutritional Value:

- Serving size: 1/2 cup

- Calories: Approximately 180

- Total fat: 14g

- Saturated fat: 10g

- Cholesterol: 0mg

- Sodium: 20mg

- Total carbohydrates: 11g

- Dietary fiber: 6g

- Sugars: 3g

- Protein: 4g

Preparation time: 5 minutes

4 - Blueberry Muffins

Ingredients:

- 1 3/4 cups all-purpose flour

- 1/2 cup granulated sugar

- 2 teaspoons baking powder

- 1/2 teaspoon salt

- 1/3 cup vegetable oil or melted butter

- 1 large egg

- 2/3 cup milk

- 1 teaspoon vanilla extract

- 1 cup fresh or frozen blueberries

Preparation:

1. Preheat your oven to 375°F (190°C) and line a muffin tin with paper liners or grease the cups lightly.

2. In a large mixing basin, whisk together the flour, sugar, baking powder, and salt.

3. In a separate bowl, whisk together the vegetable oil or melted butter, egg, milk, and vanilla extract until well combined.

4. Pour the wet ingredients into the dry ingredients and stir until just combined. Make sure not to overmix the batter; it should be lumpy.

5. Gently mix the blueberries into the batter until equally distributed.

6. Spoon the batter into the prepared muffin cups, filling them approximately two-thirds full.

7. Bake in a preheated oven for 18-20 minutes, or until a toothpick inserted into the middle of each muffin comes out clean.

8. Remove the muffins from the oven and let to cool in the pan for a few minutes before transferring to a wire rack to finish cooling.

Nutritional Value:

- Serving size: 1 muffin

- Calories: Approximately 180

- Total fat: 7g

- Saturated fat: 1g

- Cholesterol: 20mg

- Sodium: 200mg

- Total carbohydrates: 27g

- Dietary fiber: 1g

- Sugars: 11g

- Protein: 3g

Cooking Time: Approximately 18-20 minutes

5 - Cottage Pancakes

Ingredients:

- 1 cup cottage cheese

- 4 large eggs

- 1/4 cup all-purpose flour

- 2 tablespoons sugar (optional)

- 1/2 teaspoon baking powder

- 1/4 teaspoon salt

- Butter or oil for cooking

- Optional toppings: maple syrup, fresh fruit, yogurt, nuts

Preparation:

1. In a blender or food processor, combine the cottage cheese, eggs, flour, sugar (if using), baking powder, and salt. Blend until smooth.

2. Heat a non-stick skillet or griddle over medium heat and lightly grease with butter or oil.

3. Pour the batter onto the skillet or griddle to form pancakes of your desired size.

4. Cook until bubbles form on the surface of the pancakes and the edges start to look set, about 2-3 minutes.

5. Flip the pancakes and cook for an additional 1-2 minutes on the other side, until golden brown and cooked through.

6. Repeat with the remaining batter, adding more butter or oil to the skillet or griddle as needed.

7. Serve the pancakes warm with your choice of toppings, such as maple syrup, fresh fruit, yogurt, or nuts.

Nutritional Value:

- Serving size: 2 pancakes (approximately)

- Calories: Approximately 200

- Total fat: 8g

- Saturated fat: 3g

- Cholesterol: 210mg

- Sodium: 460mg

- Total carbohydrates: 14g

- Dietary fiber: 0g

- Sugars: 4g

- Protein: 17g

Cooking Time: Each pancake takes about 2-3 minutes per side, depending on the size and thickness.

6 - Greek Yogurt and Oat Pancakes

Ingredients:

- 1 cup rolled oats

- 1 cup Greek yogurt

- 2 eggs

- Two teaspoons of honey or maple syrup (optional).

- 1 teaspoon vanilla extract (optional)

- 1/2 teaspoon cinnamon (optional)

- Pinch of salt

- Cooking spray or butter for greasing the skillet

Nutritional Value (per serving, makes about 4 pancakes):

- Calories: Approximately 250g

- Protein: Approximately 15g

- Carbohydrates: Approximately 30g

- Fat: Approximately 8g

- Fiber: Approximately 3g

Preparation:

1. In a blender or food processor, combine the rolled oats, Greek yogurt, eggs, honey or maple syrup (if using), vanilla extract (if using), cinnamon (if using), and a pinch of salt.

2. Blend the mixture until smooth. If the batter is too thick, you can add a splash of milk to thin it out slightly.

3. Heat a non-stick skillet or griddle over medium heat and lightly coat it with cooking spray or butter.

4. Pour about 1/4 cup of batter onto the skillet for each pancake. Cook until bubbles develop on the pancake's surface and the edges seem firm, which should take around 2-3 minutes.

5. Flip the pancake and cook for an additional 1-2 minutes, or until golden brown and cooked through.

6. Repeat with the remaining batter, greasing the skillet as needed, Coating the Skillet if necessary.

7. Serve the pancakes warm with your favorite toppings such as fresh fruit, nuts, a drizzle of honey or maple syrup, or additional Greek yogurt.

Cooking Time: Approximately 10 minutes total (5 minutes prep, 5 minutes cooking per batch of pancakes)

7 - Apple and Pumpkin Waffles

Ingredients:

- 1 cup all-purpose flour

- 1/2 cup whole wheat flour

- 2 teaspoons baking powder

- 1/2 teaspoon baking soda

- 1/4 teaspoon salt

- 1 teaspoon ground cinnamon

- 1/2 teaspoon ground nutmeg

- 1/4 teaspoon ground ginger

- 1/4 teaspoon ground cloves

- 1 cup canned pumpkin puree

- 1 cup buttermilk

- 2 tablespoons brown sugar

- 2 large eggs, separated

- 2 tablespoons unsalted butter, melted

- 1 teaspoon vanilla extract

- 1 medium apple, peeled and grated

Preparation:

1. In a large mixing bowl, whisk together the all-purpose flour, whole wheat flour, baking powder, baking soda, salt, cinnamon, nutmeg, ginger, and cloves.

2. In another bowl, mix the pumpkin puree, buttermilk, brown sugar, egg yolks, melted butter, and vanilla extract until well combined.

3. Gradually add the wet ingredients to the dry ingredients, stirring until just combined. Fold in the grated apple.

4. In a separate clean bowl, beat the egg whites until stiff peaks form. Gently fold the beaten egg whites into the batter until just incorporated.

5. Preheat your waffle iron according to the manufacturer's instructions. Lightly grease the waffle iron with cooking spray or brush with melted butter.

6. Pour enough batter onto the preheated waffle iron to cover the waffle grid. Close the lid and cook until the waffles are golden brown and crisp about 4-5 minutes.

7. Warm the waffles with your favorite toppings such as maple syrup, whipped cream, chopped nuts, or additional grated apple.

Nutritional Value:

- **Serving Size:** This recipe makes about 4-6 waffles, depending on the size of your waffle iron.

- **Nutritional information per serving** may vary based on specific ingredients and toppings. However, each serving typically provides a good amount of fiber, vitamins A and C from the pumpkin and apple, and calcium and protein from the buttermilk and eggs.

Cooking Time:

- The cooking time for each batch of waffles will depend on your waffle iron. Generally, it takes about 4-5 minutes to cook each batch until golden brown and crisp.

8 – Buckwheat Crepes

Ingredients:

- 1 cup buckwheat flour

- 2 large eggs

- 1 1/4 cups milk (you can use cow's milk or a dairy-free alternative like almond milk)

- 1/4 teaspoon salt

- 2 tablespoons melted butter or oil (to cook in).

Optional fillings:

- For savory crêpes: cheese, ham, spinach, mushrooms, tomatoes, etc.

- For sweet crêpes: Nutella, jam, fresh fruits, whipped cream, etc.

Preparation:

1. In a large mixing bowl, whisk together the buckwheat flour and salt.

2. In a separate bowl, beat the eggs, then add them to the flour mixture.

3. Gradually pour in the milk while whisking, until you have a smooth batter.

4. Let the batter rest for at least 30 minutes to allow the flour to hydrate.

5. After resting, heat a non-stick skillet or crêpe pan over medium heat and brush it lightly with melted butter or oil.

6. Pour a small ladleful of batter into the pan, swirling it around to evenly coat the bottom.

7. Cook the crêpe for about 1-2 minutes, until the edges start to lift and the bottom is golden brown.

8. Flip the crêpe using a spatula and cook for another 1-2 minutes on the other side.

9. Repeat with the remaining batter, stacking finished crêpes on a platter as you go.

10. Once all the crêpes are cooked, fill them with your desired savory or sweet fillings, fold or roll them up, and serve immediately.

Nutritional Value (per serving, based on plain crêpes without fillings):

- Calories: Approximately 100-150

- Protein: Around 5-7 grams

- Carbohydrates: About 15-20 grams

- Fat: Roughly 3-5 grams

Cooking Time:

- Each crêpe takes about 1-2 minutes to cook on each side, so the total cooking time depends on the number of crêpes you're making. Plan for about 30-45 minutes to prepare and cook a batch of crêpes.

CHAPTER 5

Soups and Stews

1 – Kale and Tomato Soup

Ingredients:

- 1 tablespoon olive oil

- 1 medium onion, chopped

- 2 cloves garlic, minced

- 4 cups vegetable broth (or chicken broth if preferred)

- 1 can (14.5 ounces) diced tomatoes

- Two cups of chopped kale (tough stems removed).

- 1 teaspoon dried thyme

- 1/2 teaspoon dried oregano

- Salt and pepper to taste

- Grated Parmesan cheese for garnish (optional)

Preparation:

1. In a large saucepan, warm the olive oil over medium heat. Add the chopped onion and simmer for 5 minutes, or until softened.

2. Stir in the minced garlic and simmer for another 1-2 minutes, until aromatic.

3. Pour in the vegetable broth and diced tomatoes with their juices. Bring the mixture to a simmer.

4. Stir in the chopped kale, dried thyme, and dried oregano. Simmer for about 10-15 minutes, or until the kale is soft.

5. Season the soup with salt and pepper as desired.

6. Serve the soup hot, garnished with grated Parmesan cheese if desired.

Nutritional Value (per serving):

- Calories: Approximately 100-150

- Protein: Around 3-5 grams

- Carbohydrates: About 10-15 grams

- Fat: Roughly 5-7 grams

Cooking Time:

- The total cooking time for this soup is around 20-25 minutes, making it a quick and nutritious meal option.

2 - Summer Squash and Crispy

Ingredients:

- 2-3 medium summer squash (such as zucchini or yellow squash), sliced into rounds

- 1/2 cup grated Parmesan cheese

- 1/4 cup breadcrumbs

- 1/4 teaspoon garlic powder

- 1/4 teaspoon dried oregano

- Salt and pepper to taste

- 2 tablespoons olive oil

Preparation:

1. Preheat your oven to 400°F (200°C). Line a baking sheet with parchment paper or gently coat it with olive oil.

2. In a shallow bowl, mix the grated Parmesan cheese, breadcrumbs, garlic powder, dried oregano, salt, and pepper.

3. Dip each summer squash round into the olive oil, then coat it in the Parmesan mixture, pressing gently to adhere the coating to the squash.

4. Place the coated squash rounds on the prepared baking sheet in a single layer.

5. Bake in the preheated oven for about 15-20 minutes, or until the squash is tender and the Parmesan crust is crispy and golden brown.

6. Serve the crispy Parmesan-crusted summer squash hot as a delicious side dish or appetizer.

Nutritional Value (per serving):

- Calories: Approximately 100-150

- Protein: Around 4-6 grams

- Carbohydrates: About 5-8 grams

- Fat: Roughly 7-10 grams

Cooking Time: *The total cooking time for this dish is approximately 15-20 minutes*

3 - Chickpeas Soup

Ingredients:

- 2 tablespoons olive oil

- 1 large onion, chopped

- 2 cloves garlic, minced

- 2 medium carrots, diced

- 2 celery stalks, diced

- 1 teaspoon ground cumin

- 1 teaspoon ground coriander

- 1/2 teaspoon smoked paprika

- 4 cups vegetable broth (or chicken broth, if you like).

- Two cans of chickpeas (15 ounces each), drained and washed.

- 1 can (14.5 ounces) diced tomatoes

- 2 cups chopped spinach or kale

- Salt and pepper to taste

- Juice of 1 lemon

- Chopped fresh parsley for garnish (optional)

Preparation:

1. In a large saucepan, warm the olive oil over medium heat. Add the chopped onion and simmer for 5 minutes, or until softened.

2. Put the minced garlic, chopped carrots, and diced celery into the saucepan. Cook for an extra 5 minutes, turning occasionally.

3. Stir in the ground cumin, ground coriander, and smoked paprika, and cook for 1 minute until fragrant.

4. Pour in the vegetable broth, chickpeas, and diced tomatoes with their juices. Bring the mixture to a simmer.

5. Let the soup simmer for about 15-20 minutes, until the vegetables are tender and the flavors have melded together.

6. Stir in the chopped spinach or kale and cook for an additional 5 minutes, until wilted.

7. Season the soup with salt, pepper, and lemon juice to taste.

8. Serve the chickpea soup hot, garnished with chopped fresh parsley if desired.

Nutritional Value (per serving):

- Calories: Approximately 200-250

- Protein: Around 8-10 grams

- Carbohydrates: About 25-30 grams

- Fat: Roughly 7-10 grams

Cooking Time: The total cooking time for this soup is around 30-40 minutes, making it a satisfying and nutritious meal option

4 - Carrot Curry Soup

Ingredients:

- 2 tablespoons olive oil

- 1 medium onion, chopped

- 2 cloves garlic, minced

- 1 tablespoon curry powder

- 1/2 teaspoon ground cumin

- 1/2 teaspoon ground coriander

- 1/4 teaspoon ground ginger

- 4 cups vegetable broth (or chicken broth, if you like).

- 1 1/2 pounds peeled and diced carrots.

- 1 can (14 ounces) coconut milk

- Salt and pepper to taste

- Juice of 1 lime

- Chopped fresh cilantro for garnish (optional)

Preparation:

1. In a large saucepan, warm the olive oil over medium heat. Add the chopped onion and simmer for 5 minutes, or until softened.

2. Add the minced garlic, curry powder, ground cumin, ground coriander, and ground ginger to the pot. Prepare for another 1-2 minutes, until fragrant.

3. Pour in the vegetable broth and add the chopped carrots. Bring the mixture to a simmer and cook for about 15-20 minutes, until the carrots are tender.

4. Using an immersion blender or regular blender, puree the soup until smooth.

5. Stir in the coconut milk and continue to cook for another 5 minutes, until heated through.

6. Season the soup with salt, pepper, and lime juice to taste.

7. Serve the carrot curry soup hot, garnished with chopped fresh cilantro if desired.

Nutritional Value (per serving):

- Calories: Approximately 200-250

- Protein: Around 2-4 grams

- Carbohydrates: About 15-20 grams

- Fat: Roughly 15-20 grams

Cooking Time: The total cooking time for this soup is around 25-30 minutes. It's a flavorful and comforting dish, perfect for chilly days.

5 - Lamb and Vegetable Stew

Ingredients:

- 1 1/2 pounds lamb stew meat, cut into bite-sized pieces

- 2 tablespoons olive oil

- 1 medium onion, chopped

- 2 cloves garlic, minced

- 2 medium carrots, diced

- 2 stalks celery, diced

- 2 medium potatoes, peeled and diced

- 1 can (14.5 ounces) diced tomatoes

- 4 cups beef or lamb broth

- 1 teaspoon dried thyme

- 1 teaspoon dried rosemary

- Salt and pepper to taste

- 1 cup frozen peas

- Chopped fresh parsley for garnish (optional)

Preparation:

1. Warm the olive oil in a big saucepan or Dutch oven over medium heat. Add the lamb stew meat and cook until browned on all sides, about 5-7 minutes.

2. Remove the lamb from the saucepan and put it aside. Cook the chopped onion until softened, approximately 5 minutes.

3. Add the minced garlic, diced carrots, diced celery, and diced potatoes to the pot. Cook for an extra 5 minutes, stirring occasionally.

4. Return the browned lamb to the pot. Pour in the diced tomatoes with their juices and the beef or lamb broth.

5. Stir in the dried thyme and dried rosemary. Mix the stew with salt and pepper, to taste.

6. Bring the stew to a simmer, then reduce the heat to low and cover. Let the stew simmer for about 1 1/2 to 2 hours, stirring occasionally, until the lamb is tender.

7. Stir in the frozen peas during the last 10 minutes of cooking.

8. Taste and adjust seasoning as required.

9. Serve the lamb and vegetable stew hot, garnished with chopped fresh parsley if desired.

Nutritional Value (per serving):

- Calories: Approximately 300-400

- Protein: Around 25-30 grams

- Carbohydrates: About 20-25 grams

- Fat: Roughly 15-20 grams

Cooking Time: The total cooking time for this stew is around 2 to 2 1/2 hours

6 – Beef, Mushroom, and Pearl Barley Soup

Ingredients:

- 1 pound beef stew meat, cubed

- 2 tablespoons olive oil

- 1 medium onion, chopped

- 2 cloves garlic, minced

- 8 ounces mushrooms, sliced

- 2 medium carrots, diced

- 2 stalks celery, diced

- 1 cup pearl barley

- 6 cups beef broth

- 1 teaspoon dried thyme

- 1 teaspoon dried rosemary

- Salt and pepper to taste

- Chopped fresh parsley for garnish (optional)

Preparation:

1. In a large saucepan or Dutch oven, warm the olive oil over medium heat. Cook the beef stew meat until browned on both sides, approximately 5-7 minutes. Remove the steak from the saucepan and put it aside.

2. Cook the chopped onion in the saucepan until softened, approximately 5 minutes. Add the minced garlic and simmer for another 1-2 minutes, or until fragrant.

3. Add the sliced mushrooms to the pot and cook until they release their juices and start to brown, about 5-7 minutes.

4. Return the browned beef to the pot. Add the diced carrots, diced celery, pearl barley, beef broth, dried thyme, and dried rosemary.

5. Bring the soup to a simmer, then reduce the heat to low and cover. Let the soup simmer for about 45 minutes to 1 hour, until the beef is tender and the barley is cooked through.

6. Season the soup with salt and pepper, to taste.

7. Serve the beef, mushroom, and pearl barley soup hot, garnished with chopped fresh parsley if desired.

Nutritional Value (per serving):

- Calories: Approximately 300-400

- Protein: Around 20-25 grams

- Carbohydrates: About 25-30 grams

- Fat: Roughly 10-15 grams

Cooking Time: The total cooking time for this soup is approximately 1 to 1 1/2 hours

7 - Cheesy Chicken Tortilla Soup

Ingredients:

- 1 tablespoon olive oil

- 1 medium onion, chopped

- 2 cloves garlic, minced

- Optional: 1 diced jalapeño pepper with seeds.

- 1 teaspoon ground cumin

- 1 teaspoon chili powder

- 1 can (14.5 ounces) diced tomatoes

- 4 cups chicken broth

- 2 cups cooked shredded chicken

- 1 cup frozen corn kernels.

- 1 canned (15 ounce) black beans, drained and rinsed.

- 1 cup shredded cheddar cheese

- 1/4 cup chopped fresh cilantro

- Juice of 1 lime

- Salt and pepper to taste

- Tortilla strips or chips for serving

- Additional shredded cheese, sour cream, avocado slices, and lime wedges for garnish (optional)

Preparation:

1. In a big saucepan, bring the olive oil to medium heat. Add the chopped onion and simmer for 5 minutes, or until softened.

2. Add the minced garlic and diced jalapeño pepper (if using) to the pot, and cook for another 1-2 minutes until fragrant.

3. Stir in the ground cumin and chili powder, and cook for 1 minute.

4. Pour in the diced tomatoes with their juices and the chicken broth. Bring the mixture to a simmer.

5. Add the shredded chicken, frozen corn kernels, and black beans to the pot. Allow the soup to boil for 15-20 minutes to merge the flavors.

6. Stir in the shredded cheddar cheese, chopped fresh cilantro, and lime juice. Season the soup with salt and pepper, to taste.

7. Serve the cheesy chicken tortilla soup hot, garnished with tortilla strips or chips, and additional shredded cheese, sour cream, avocado slices, and lime wedges if desired.

Nutritional Value (per serving):

- Calories: Approximately 300-400

- Protein: Around 20-25 grams

-   Carbohydrates: About 20-25 grams

-   Fat: Roughly 15-20 grams

Cooking Time: The total cooking time for this soup is approximately 30-40 minutes

CHAPTER 6

Salads

1 - Summer Salad with Honey Dressing

Ingredients:

- Mixed salad greens (such as lettuce, spinach, and arugula).

- Cherry tomatoes, halved

- Cucumber, sliced

- Red onion, thinly sliced

- Avocado, sliced

- Feta cheese, crumbled

- Walnuts or almonds, toasted (optional)

For the Honey Dressing:

- 3 tablespoons olive oil

- 2 tablespoons apple cider vinegar

- 1 tablespoon honey

- 1 teaspoon Dijon mustard

- Salt and pepper to taste

Instructions:

1. In a small bowl, mix the olive oil, apple cider vinegar, honey, Dijon mustard, salt, and pepper. Set aside.

2. In a large salad bowl, combine the mixed salad greens, cherry tomatoes, cucumber, red onion, avocado, and feta cheese.

3. Drizzle the honey dressing over the salad and toss gently to coat.

4. If using, sprinkle toasted walnuts or almonds on top.

5. Serve immediately and enjoy your refreshing summer salad!

2 - Cucumber and Kidney Bean Salad

Ingredients:

- 1 cucumber, diced

- Drain and rinse 1 can (15 oz) of kidney beans.

- 1/4 cup red onion, finely chopped

- 1/4 cup fresh parsley, chopped

- 2 tablespoons olive oil

- 2 tablespoons apple cider vinegar

- 1 teaspoon honey

- Salt and pepper to taste

Instructions:

1. In a large bowl, combine the diced cucumber, kidney beans, chopped red onion, and fresh parsley.

2. In a small bowl, whisk together the olive oil, apple cider vinegar, honey, salt, and pepper to make the dressing.

3. Pour the dressing over the cucumber and kidney bean mixture, and toss gently to coat everything evenly.

4. Taste and adjust seasoning if necessary.

5. Refrigerate the salad for at least 30 minutes to enable the flavors to come together.

6. Serve chilled as a side dish or a light meal option.

3 - Sofrito Steak and Veg Salad

Ingredients:

For the steak:

- 1 lb flank steak

- 2 tablespoons olive oil

- 2 tablespoons sofrito sauce (store-bought or homemade)

- Salt and pepper to taste

For the salad:

- Mixed salad greens (such as spinach, arugula, and lettuce)

- Cherry tomatoes, halved

- Red bell pepper, sliced

- Red onion, thinly sliced

- Avocado, sliced

- Feta cheese, crumbled

For the dressing:

- 1/4 cup olive oil

- 2 tablespoons red wine vinegar

- 1 tablespoon lime juice

- 1 teaspoon honey

- 1 clove garlic, minced

- Salt and pepper to taste

Instructions:

1. Marinate the steak: In a bowl, mix the olive oil, sofrito sauce, salt, and pepper. Rub the mixture over the flank steak, ensuring it's evenly coated. Allow to marinate for at least 30 minutes, preferably overnight in the refrigerator for optimum flavor.

2. Cook the steak: Heat a grill or grill pan over medium-high heat. Cook the steak for 4-5 minutes on each side for medium-rare, or until desired doneness. Remove from heat and let it rest for a few minutes before slicing thinly against the grain.

3. Prepare the salad: In a large salad bowl, combine the mixed salad greens, cherry tomatoes, red bell pepper, red onion, avocado, and feta cheese.

4. Make the dressing: In a small bowl, whisk together the olive oil, red wine vinegar, lime juice, honey, minced garlic, salt, and pepper until well combined.

5. Assemble the salad: Arrange the sliced steak over the salad mixture.

6. Drizzle the dressing over the salad and steak.

7. Toss gently to combine, ensuring everything is evenly coated with the dressing.

8. Serve immediately and enjoy your flavorful Sofrito Steak and Veg Salad!

4 - Black Rice and Edamame Salad

Ingredients:

For the salad:

- 1 cup black rice

- 1 1/2 cups shelled edamame, fresh or frozen.

- 1 red bell pepper, diced

- 1/2 cup shredded carrots

- 1/4 cup chopped green onions

- 1/4 cup chopped fresh cilantro

- 1/4 cup sliced almonds, toasted

- Optional: sesame seeds for garnish

For the dressing:

- 3 tablespoons rice vinegar

- 2 tablespoons soy sauce

- 1 tablespoon sesame oil

- 1 tablespoon honey or maple syrup

- 1 clove garlic, minced

- 1 teaspoon grated ginger

- Salt and pepper to taste

Instructions:

1. Cook the black rice according to package instructions. Once cooked, let it cool to room temperature.

2. Cook the edamame in boiling water for about 3-5 minutes, or until tender. To halt the cooking

process, drain and rinse well with cold water. Set aside.

3. In a large bowl, combine the cooked black rice, cooked edamame, diced red bell pepper, shredded carrots, chopped green onions, chopped cilantro, and toasted sliced almonds.

4. In a small bowl, whisk together the rice vinegar, soy sauce, sesame oil, honey or maple syrup, minced garlic, grated ginger, salt, and pepper to make the dressing.

5. Pour the dressing over the salad ingredients in a large bowl.

6. Toss the salad gently until everything is well coated with the dressing.

7. Taste and adjust seasoning, if necessary, with more salt, pepper, or vinegar.

8. Garnish with sesame seeds, if desired.

9. Serve chilled or at room temperature as a delicious and nutritious side dish or light meal option.

5 - Farro and Strawberry Salad

Ingredients:

For the salad:

- 1 cup farro

- 2 cups water or vegetable broth

- 2 cups fresh strawberries, sliced

- 1/2 cup crumbled feta cheese

- 1/4 cup chopped fresh basil leaves

- 1/4 cup chopped fresh mint leaves

- 1/4 cup sliced almonds, toasted

For the dressing:

- 3 tablespoons balsamic vinegar

- 2 tablespoons extra virgin olive oil

- 1 tablespoon honey or maple syrup

- Salt and pepper to taste

Instructions:

1. Rinse the farro under cold water. In a medium saucepan, combine the rinsed farro and water or vegetable broth. Bring to a boil, then reduce the heat to low, cover, and simmer for about 25-30 minutes, or until the farro is tender but still chewy. Drain any extra liquid and chill the farro to room temperature.

2. In a small bowl, whisk together the balsamic vinegar, olive oil, honey or maple syrup, salt, and pepper to make the dressing. Set aside.

3. In a large salad bowl, combine the cooked farro, sliced strawberries, crumbled feta cheese, chopped basil, and chopped mint.

4. Pour the dressing over the salad ingredients in a large bowl.

5. Toss the salad gently until everything is well coated with the dressing.

6. Sprinkle the toasted sliced almonds over the salad as a garnish.

7. Taste and adjust seasoning, if necessary, with more salt, pepper, or vinegar.

8. Serve chilled or at room temperature as a refreshing and flavorful side dish or light meal option.

6 - Cobb Salad

Ingredients:

For the salad:

- 4 cups mixed salad greens (such as lettuce, spinach, and arugula)

- 2 cooked chicken breasts, diced

- 4 hard-boiled eggs, sliced

- 6 slices cooked bacon, crumbled

- 1 cup cherry tomatoes, halved

- 1 avocado, diced

- 1/2 cup crumbled blue cheese or feta cheese

- 1/4 cup sliced green onions

- Optional: sliced cucumber, sliced radishes

For the dressing:

- 1/4 cup extra virgin olive oil

- 2 tablespoons red wine vinegar

- 1 tablespoon Dijon mustard

- 1 teaspoon honey or maple syrup

- Salt and pepper to taste

Instructions:

1. Begin with the mixed salad greens in a large salad bowl.

2. Arrange the diced cooked chicken, sliced hard-boiled eggs, crumbled bacon, cherry tomatoes, diced avocado, crumbled blue cheese, and sliced green onions in rows over the salad greens.

3. If using, add sliced cucumber and sliced radishes for extra crunch and flavor.

4. In a small bowl, whisk together the extra virgin olive oil, red wine vinegar, Dijon mustard, honey or maple syrup, salt, and pepper to make the dressing.

5. Drizzle the dressing on the Cobb Salad.

6. Serve immediately, allowing each person to toss their salad with the dressing to their preference, or serve the dressing on the side.

7 - Kale, Cantaloupe, and Chicken Salad

Ingredients:

For the salad:

- 4 cups mixed salad greens (such as lettuce, spinach, and arugula)

- 2 cooked chicken breasts, diced

- 4 hard-boiled eggs, sliced

- 6 slices cooked bacon, crumbled

- 1 cup cherry tomatoes, halved

- 1 avocado, diced

- 1/2 cup crumbled blue cheese or feta cheese

- 1/4 cup sliced green onions

- Optional: sliced cucumber, sliced radishes

For the dressing:

- 1/4 cup extra virgin olive oil

- 2 tablespoons red wine vinegar

- 1 tablespoon Dijon mustard

- 1 teaspoon honey or maple syrup

- Salt and pepper to taste

Instructions:

1. Begin with the mixed salad greens in a large salad bowl.

2. Arrange the diced cooked chicken, sliced hard-boiled eggs, crumbled bacon, cherry tomatoes, diced avocado, crumbled blue cheese, and sliced green onions in rows over the salad greens.

3. If using, add sliced cucumber and sliced radishes for extra crunch and flavor.

4. In a small bowl, whisk together the extra virgin olive oil, red wine vinegar, Dijon mustard, honey or maple syrup, salt, and pepper to make the dressing.

5. Drizzle the dressing on the Cobb Salad.

6. Serve immediately, allowing each person to toss their salad with the dressing to their preference, or serve the dressing on the side.

CHAPTER 7

Snacks and Appetizers

1. Easy Cauliflower Hush Puppies

Ingredients:

- 1 head cauliflower, chopped into florets

- 1 cup cornmeal

- 1/4 cup all-purpose flour

- 2 eggs

- 1/4 cup chopped green onions

- 1/4 cup shredded cheddar cheese

- 1 teaspoon garlic powder

- Salt and pepper to taste

- Vegetable oil for frying

Preparation:

1. Cook the cauliflower florets in boiling water for 5-7 minutes until tender. Drain and mash.

2. In a bowl, combine the mashed cauliflower with cornmeal, flour, eggs, green onions, cheddar cheese, garlic powder, salt, and pepper.

3. Heat vegetable oil in a frying pan over medium heat. Drop spoonful of the cauliflower mixture into the hot oil and fry until golden brown, about 3-4 minutes per side.

4. Remove from oil and drain on paper towels. Serve hot.

Nutritional Value:

- Calories: 150 per serving

- Protein: 5g

- Carbohydrates: 20g

- Fat: 6g

Cooking Time: 20 minutes

2. Parmesan Crisps

Ingredients:

- 1 cup grated Parmesan cheese.

Preparation:

1. Preheat oven to 400°F (200°C). Line the baking sheet with parchment paper.

2. Place small mounds of grated Parmesan cheese on the prepared baking sheet, spacing them a few inches apart.

3. Flatten each mound slightly with the back of a spoon.

4. Bake in the preheated oven for 5-7 minutes, until golden and crisp.

5. Remove from oven and let cool completely before serving.

Nutritional Value:

- Calories: 80 per serving

- Protein: 7g

- Carbohydrates: 1g

- Fat: 5g

Cooking Time: 10 minutes

3. Cauliflower Mash

Ingredients:

- 1 head cauliflower, chopped into florets

- 2 cloves garlic, minced

- 2 tablespoons butter

- 1/4 cup grated Parmesan cheese

- Salt and pepper to taste

- Chopped chives or parsley for garnish (optional)

Preparation:

1. Steam or boil the cauliflower florets and minced garlic until tender, about 10-12 minutes.

2. Drain the cauliflower and garlic, then transfer to a food processor or blender.

3. Add butter, Parmesan cheese, salt, and pepper to the cauliflower mixture.

4. Blend until smooth and creamy.

5. Adjust seasoning if necessary, then transfer to a serving dish.

6. Garnish with chopped chives or parsley if desired.

Nutritional Value:

- Calories: 120 per serving

- Protein: 5g

- Carbohydrates: 8g

- Fat: 8g

Cooking Time: 15 minutes

4. Banana and Carrot Flax Muffins:

Ingredients:

- 2 ripe bananas, mashed

- 1 cup grated carrots

- 2 eggs

- 1/4 cup maple syrup or honey.

- 1/4 cup melted coconut oil

- 1 teaspoon vanilla extract

- 1 cup almond flour

- 1/4 cup ground flaxseed

- 1 teaspoon baking powder

- 1/2 teaspoon ground cinnamon

- Pinch of salt

Preparation:

1. Preheat oven to 350°F (175°C). Line the muffin tray with paper liners.

2. In a large bowl, mix together mashed bananas, grated carrots, eggs, honey or maple syrup, melted coconut oil, and vanilla extract.

3. In a separate bowl, combine almond flour, ground flaxseed, baking powder, cinnamon, and salt.

4. Gradually incorporate the dry ingredients into the wet components, stirring until completely blended.

5. Spoon the batter into the prepared muffin tin, filling each cup about 2/3 full.

6. Bake in a preheated oven for 20-25 minutes, or until a toothpick inserted into the middle of each muffin comes out clean.

7. Remove from the oven and let it cool in the pan for 5 minutes before transferring to a wire rack to finish cooling.

Nutritional Value:

- Calories: 180 per muffin

- Protein: 4g

- Carbohydrates: 18g

- Fat: 11g

Cooking Time: 25 minutes

5. Easy Low-Carb Biscuits

Ingredients:

- 2 cups almond flour

- 1/4 cup coconut flour

- 2 teaspoons baking powder

- 1/2 teaspoon garlic powder

- 1/4 teaspoon salt

- 1/2 cup unsalted butter, melted

- 2 large eggs

-   1/4 cup Greek yogurt or sour cream.

Preparation:

1. Preheat oven to 350°F (175°C). Line the baking sheet with parchment paper.

2. In a large bowl, whisk together almond flour, coconut flour, baking powder, garlic powder, and salt.

3. In a separate bowl, mix together melted butter, eggs, sour cream or Greek yogurt.

4. Gradually combine the wet and dry ingredients, stirring until a dough forms.

5. Divide the dough into equal portions and shape into biscuits.

6. Place the biscuits on the prepared baking sheet and flatten slightly with your hand.

7. Bake in the preheated oven for 12-15 minutes, or until golden brown.

8. Remove from oven and let cool slightly before serving.

Nutritional Value:

- Calories: 180 per biscuit

- Protein: 6g

- Carbohydrates: 5g

- Fat: 16g

Cooking Time: 15 minutes

6. Zucchini and Banana Bread

Ingredients:

- 2 ripe bananas, mashed

- 1 cup shredded zucchini, squeezed to remove excess moisture.

- Use 1/4 cup melted coconut or vegetable oil.

- 1/4 cup honey or maple syrup.

- 2 eggs

- 1 teaspoon vanilla extract

- 1 1/2 cups almond flour

- 1/4 cup coconut flour

- 1 teaspoon baking powder

- 1/2 teaspoon baking soda

- 1/2 teaspoon ground cinnamon

- Pinch of salt

- If desired, add chopped nuts or chocolate chips.

Preparation:

1. Preheat oven to 350°F (175°C). Grease a 9x5-inch loaf pan.

2. In a large bowl, mix together mashed bananas, shredded zucchini, melted coconut oil or vegetable oil, honey or maple syrup, eggs, and vanilla extract.

3. In a separate bowl, whisk together almond flour, coconut flour, baking powder, baking soda, cinnamon, and salt.

4. Gradually incorporate the dry ingredients into the wet components, stirring until completely blended.

5. Fold in chopped nuts or chocolate chips if using.

6. Pour the batter into the prepared loaf pan and spread evenly.

7. Bake in a preheated oven for 50-60 minutes, or until a toothpick inserted in the middle comes out clean.

8. Remove from oven and let cool in the pan for 10 minutes before transferring to a wire rack to cool completely.

Nutritional Value:

- Calories: 200 per slice (assuming 12 slices)

- Protein: 6g

-   Carbohydrates: 18g

-   Fat: 12g

Cooking Time: 60 minutes

CHAPTER 8

Desserts

1. Peanut Butter and Pineapple Smoothie

Ingredients:

- One cup of frozen pineapple chunks.

- 2 tablespoons of peanut butter

- 1 banana

- 1 cup of almond milk

Preparation:

1. Combine all ingredients in a blender.

2. Blend until smooth.

3. Fill a glass and serve immediately.

Nutritional Value:

- Calories: Approx. 300

- Protein: 8g

- Fat: 12g

- Carbohydrates: 40g

- Fiber: 6g

Cooking Time:

- Preparation time: 5 minutes

- No cooking required

2. Peach, Banana, and Almond Pancakes

Ingredients:

- 1 ripe banana, mashed

- 1 peach, diced

- 1 cup almond flour

- 2 eggs

- 1/2 teaspoon baking powder

- Pinch of salt

- Almond milk (as required for consistency).

Preparation:

1. In a bowl, mix mashed banana, diced peach, almond flour, eggs, baking powder, and salt.

2. Add almond milk gradually until you achieve a pancake batter consistency.

3. Heat a non-stick pan over medium heat and pour batter onto the pan.

4. Cook until bubbles form on the surface, then flip and cook until golden brown on both sides.

Nutritional Value:

-   Calories: Approx. 200 per pancake

-   Protein: 8g

-   Fat: 12g

-   Carbohydrates: 18g

-   Fiber: 4g

Cooking Time:

- Preparation time: 10 minutes

- Cooking time: 10 minutes

3. Apple Cinnamon Chimichanga

Ingredients:

- 2 large flour tortillas

- 2 apples, peeled and diced

- 2 tablespoons sugar

- 1 teaspoon cinnamon

- Cooking oil for frying

Preparation:

1. In a bowl, mix diced apples with sugar and cinnamon.

2. Place apple mixture onto the center of each tortilla.

3. Fold the sides of the tortillas over the filling and roll them up.

4. Heat oil in a pan and fry the chimichangas until golden brown.

5. Remove from oil and drain excess oil on paper towels.

Nutritional Value:

- Calories: Approx. 300 per Chimichanga

- Protein: 2g

- Fat: 12g

- Carbohydrates: 45g

- Fiber: 6g

Cooking Time:

- Preparation time: 15 minutes

- Cooking time: 5 minutes

4. Chia and Raspberry Pudding

Ingredients:

- 1/4 cup chia seeds

- 1 cup almond milk

- Use 1 tablespoon of honey or maple syrup.

- 1/2 cup raspberries

Preparation:

1. In a bowl, mix chia seeds, almond milk, and honey/maple syrup.

2. Let it sit in the refrigerator for at least 2 hours or overnight, stirring occasionally.

3. Once the mixture has thickened to a pudding-like consistency, stir in raspberries.

4. Serve chilled.

Nutritional Value:

- Calories: Approx. 150 per serving

- Protein: 5g

- Fat: 8g

- Carbohydrates: 15g

- Fiber: 10g

Cooking Time:

- Preparation time: 5 minutes

- Refrigerate for 2 hours or overnight.

5. Crispy Apple Chips

Ingredients:

- 2 apples, thinly sliced

- 1 teaspoon cinnamon

- Cooking spray

Preparation:

1. Preheat oven to 200°F (93°C).

2. Place thinly sliced apples on a baking sheet lined with parchment paper.

3. Sprinkle cinnamon over the apple slices.

4. Lightly coat with cooking spray.

5. Bake in the preheated oven for 1.5 to 2 hours, or until the chips are crispy.

6. Allow to cool before serving.

Nutritional Value:

- Calories: Approx. 50 per serving (depending on the size of the apples)

- Protein: 0g

- Fat: 0g

- Carbohydrates: 15g

- Fiber: 3g

Cooking Time:

- Preparation time: 10 minutes

- Baking time is 1.5 to 2 hours.

6. Easy Banana Mug Cake

Ingredients:

- 1 ripe banana, mashed

- 1 egg

- 2 tablespoons almond flour

- 1/2 teaspoon baking powder

- Optional: 1 tablespoon honey or maple syrup

Preparation:

1. In a microwave-safe mug, mix mashed banana, egg, almond flour, and baking powder.

2. If desired, add honey or maple syrup for sweetness.

3. Microwave on high for 2-3 minutes, or until the cake is set.

4. Let it cool for a minute before enjoying it.

Nutritional Value:

- Calories: Approx. 200 per serving

- Protein: 7g

- Fat: 8g

- Carbohydrates: 25g

- Fiber: 4g

Cooking Time:

- Preparation time: 5 minutes

- Cooking time: 2-3 minutes in the microwave.

CONCLUSION

"The Complete Diabetic Cookbook for Beginners 2024" provides a wide range of tasty and healthy dishes designed exclusively for people with diabetes. With a focus on balanced ingredients and mindful cooking methods, this cookbook empowers readers to take control of their health while enjoying flavorful meals.

Each recipe within this cookbook is carefully crafted to meet the dietary needs of individuals with diabetes, providing clear instructions, precise ingredient measurements, and comprehensive nutritional information. From vibrant smoothies to hearty pancakes, from crunchy snacks to indulgent desserts, there's something for every palate and occasion.

By incorporating wholesome ingredients such as fruits, vegetables, lean proteins, and whole grains, these recipes not only help regulate blood sugar levels but also support overall well-being. With an emphasis on portion control and mindful eating, readers can feel confident in making informed choices about their nutrition without sacrificing taste or satisfaction.

Beyond the kitchen, "The Complete Diabetic Cookbook for Beginners 2024" serves as a valuable resource for individuals seeking to improve their health and manage their condition proactively. It offers practical tips on meal planning, grocery shopping, and dining out, empowering readers to navigate various social and culinary situations with confidence and ease.

In conclusion, this cookbook is more than just a collection of recipes—it's a guide to living well with diabetes. By embracing the principles of balanced nutrition, portion control, and mindful eating, readers can not only manage their condition effectively but also thrive and enjoy a vibrant, fulfilling life.

As you embark on your journey with "The Complete Diabetic Cookbook for Beginners 2024," remember that every meal is an opportunity to nourish your body and nurture your health. By embracing these delicious and wholesome recipes, you're not just making dietary changes; you're committing yourself—to prioritize your well-being and savor the joys of good food. So let this cookbook be your companion on the path to better health, one delicious dish at a time. You deserve it.

BONUS

21-Days Meal Plan

Day 1:

- Breakfast: Scrambled eggs with spinach and tomatoes, whole grain toast

- Lunch: Grilled chicken salad with mixed greens, cucumbers, and vinaigrette dressing

- Dinner: Baked salmon with quinoa and steamed broccoli

- Snacks: Greek yogurt with berries

Day 2:

- Breakfast: Oatmeal with sliced almonds and strawberries

- Lunch: Turkey wrap with whole wheat tortilla, lettuce, and avocado

- Dinner: Vegetable stir-fry with tofu and brown rice

- Snacks: Carrot sticks with hummus

Day 3:

- Breakfast: Greek yogurt parfait with granola and sliced peaches

- Lunch: Lentil soup with a side of mixed green salad

- Dinner: Grilled shrimp with roasted sweet potatoes and asparagus

- Snacks: Apple slices with peanut butter.

Day 4:

- Breakfast: Whole grain toast with avocado and poached eggs

- Lunch: Quinoa salad with chickpeas, cherry tomatoes, and feta cheese

- Dinner: Baked chicken breast with roasted Brussels sprouts and quinoa

- Snacks: Cottage cheese with pineapple chunks

Day 5:

- Breakfast: Smoothie made with spinach, banana, almond milk, and protein powder

- Lunch: Grilled vegetable wrap with hummus in a whole wheat tortilla

- Dinner: Turkey meatballs with whole wheat spaghetti and marinara sauce

- Snacks: Edamame

Day 6:

- Breakfast: Whole grain waffles with Greek yogurt and mixed berries

- Lunch: Tuna salad with mixed greens, bell peppers, and balsamic vinaigrette

- Dinner: Baked cod with steamed brown rice and green beans

- Snacks: Almonds and dried apricots.

Day 7:

- Breakfast: Veggie omelet with mushrooms, bell peppers, and onions

- Lunch: Quinoa and black bean salad with avocado and lime vinaigrette

- Dinner: Grilled steak with roasted sweet potato wedges and asparagus

- Snacks: Celery sticks with almond butter.

Day 8:

- Breakfast: Cottage cheese pancakes with mixed berries

- Lunch: Chicken Caesar salad with romaine lettuce, grilled chicken breast, and light Caesar dressing

- Dinner: Vegetable curry with tofu and brown rice

- Snacks: Cherry tomatoes with mozzarella cheese

Day 9:

- Breakfast: Whole grain toast with almond butter and sliced banana

- Lunch: Lentil and vegetable stew with a side of whole grain bread

- Dinner: Baked tilapia with quinoa pilaf and steamed broccoli

- Snacks: Air-popped popcorn seasoned with a sprinkle of Parmesan cheese

Day 10:

- Breakfast: Egg muffins with spinach, bell peppers, and feta cheese

- Lunch: Spinach and feta stuffed chicken breast with a side of roasted sweet potatoes

- Dinner: Turkey chili with kidney beans and a side of whole grain cornbread

- Snacks: Cottage cheese with sliced cucumber

Day 11:

- Breakfast: Overnight oats with chia seeds, almond milk, and sliced peaches

- Lunch: Mediterranean quinoa salad with cherry tomatoes, cucumbers, olives, and feta cheese

- Dinner: Grilled vegetable kebabs with tofu and quinoa

- Snacks: Sliced bell peppers with guacamole

Day 12:

- Breakfast: Whole grain English muffin with scrambled eggs and avocado

- Lunch: Asian-inspired chicken salad with cabbage, carrots, and sesame ginger dressing

- Dinner: Baked cod with roasted Brussels sprouts and wild rice

- Snacks: Greek yogurt with a drizzle of honey

Day 13:

- Breakfast: Smoothie bowl topped with granola, sliced almonds, and mixed berries

- Lunch: Turkey and avocado wrap with whole wheat tortilla, lettuce, and tomato

- Dinner: Stir-fried tofu with mixed vegetables and brown rice

- Snacks: Apple slices with cinnamon

Day 14:

- Breakfast: Whole grain pancakes with Greek yogurt and sliced strawberries

- Lunch: Quinoa and black bean wrap with avocado, lettuce, and salsa

- Dinner: Grilled chicken breast with roasted sweet potatoes and green beans

- Snacks: Celery sticks with cream cheese and smoked salmon.

Day 15:

- Breakfast: Veggie-packed omelet with mushrooms, spinach, and cherry tomatoes

- Lunch: Chickpea and vegetable salad with a lemon tahini dressing

- Dinner: Baked salmon with quinoa and steamed asparagus

- Snacks: Mixed nuts and dried cranberries

Day 16:

- Breakfast: Whole grain toast with mashed avocado
  and poached eggs

- Lunch: Spinach and grilled chicken salad with
  strawberries and balsamic vinaigrette

- Dinner: Turkey burgers on whole wheat buns with
  sweet potato fries

- Snacks: Carrot and cucumber sticks with hummus

Day 17:

- Breakfast: Greek yogurt with granola and sliced
  peaches

- Lunch: Lentil soup with a side of mixed greens
  and vinaigrette

- Dinner: Baked cod with quinoa pilaf and roasted
  vegetables

- Snacks: Cottage cheese with pineapple chunks

Day 18:

- Breakfast: Smoothie made with spinach, banana, almond milk, and protein powder

- Lunch: Turkey and avocado wrap with whole wheat tortilla, lettuce, and tomato

- Dinner: Grilled tofu with stir-fried vegetables and brown rice

- Snacks: Edamame sprinkled with sea salt

Day 19:

- Breakfast: Whole grain waffles with Greek yogurt and mixed berries

- Lunch: Quinoa salad with black beans, corn, avocado, and lime vinaigrette

- Dinner: Chicken stir-fry with broccoli, bell peppers, and snap peas over brown rice

- Snacks: Almonds and dried apricots

Day 20:

- Breakfast: Veggie scramble with eggs, bell peppers, onions, and spinach

- Lunch: Caprese salad with tomatoes, mozzarella, basil, and balsamic glaze

- Dinner: Grilled shrimp skewers with quinoa and roasted vegetables

- Snacks: Celery sticks with almond butter and raisins

Day 21:

- Breakfast: Overnight oats with almond milk, chia seeds, and sliced bananas

- Lunch: Mediterranean quinoa salad with cucumbers, olives, feta cheese, and lemon vinaigrette

- Dinner: Baked chicken breast with roasted sweet potatoes and steamed broccoli

- Snacks: Sliced apple with peanut butter

www.ingramcontent.com/pod-product-compliance
Lightning Source LLC
Chambersburg PA
CBHW070758260726
48660CB00005B/1674